Home Workout Hero

Andy Clarke

Published by works, 2023.

HOME WORKOUT HERO

First edition. October 23, 2023.

Copyright © 2023 Andy Clarke.

ISBN: 979-8223011064

Written by Andy Clarke.

Table of Contents

The Benefits of Home Workouts

Home workouts have gained tremendous popularity in recent years, and for good reason. The benefits of exercising in the comfort of your own home are numerous and can positively impact various aspects of your physical and mental well-being.

One of the most significant advantages of home workouts is the unparalleled convenience they offer. With no need for a commute to the gym, you save valuable time that can be used for the workout itself or other essential daily tasks. This flexibility in scheduling allows you to integrate exercise seamlessly into your daily routine, making it more likely that you'll stick to your fitness goals. Whether you're an early bird who enjoys morning workouts or prefer late-night sessions, the choice is entirely yours.

Cost-effectiveness is another compelling reason to opt for home workouts. While gyms often require ongoing membership fees, home workouts typically entail a one-time or occasional investment in fitness equipment or apps. Over time, this can translate into significant savings, making it an attractive option for those on a budget.

The privacy and comfort of home workouts also play a crucial role in motivating individuals. Exercising in a judgment-free environment without the presence of others can reduce self-consciousness and boost self-esteem. This sense of privacy encourages people to explore different forms of exercise, ultimately contributing to a more diversified and enjoyable fitness routine.

Flexibility is a defining feature of home workouts. You have the freedom to choose the exercises, duration, and intensity that best suit your preferences and fitness goals. There's no need to adhere to a set class schedule or share equipment with others, which can often be a source of frustration in crowded gyms. Whether you're following online workout videos, practicing yoga, doing high-intensity interval training, or lifting weights, the options are virtually limitless.

Moreover, home workouts accommodate individuals of all fitness levels and physical conditions. Beginners can start at their own pace and gradually build strength and endurance, while advanced athletes can tailor workouts to challenge themselves continually. The adaptability of home workouts is further enhanced by the ability to create a personalized workout environment, adjusting factors like temperature, lighting, and music to foster motivation and focus.

In these times of uncertainty, home workouts also offer a degree of resilience. Regardless of external factors such as extreme weather conditions, public health concerns, or the availability of gym facilities, your home remains a consistent and dependable fitness haven.

In summary, home workouts are a versatile and empowering option for maintaining a healthy and active lifestyle. They provide unparalleled convenience, save you money, and offer privacy and comfort. This flexibility, accessibility, and adaptability, combined with the ability to create a personalized workout environment, make home workouts an attractive choice for individuals seeking a sustainable and effective fitness routine.

Setting Up Your Home Gym

Setting up my home gym has been a rewarding project that's brought a significant positive change to my fitness routine. It all started with selecting the right space within my home. I opted for an area with sufficient natural light, good ventilation, and enough space to accommodate my fitness equipment without feeling cramped. The choice of location plays a pivotal role in creating an inviting workout environment, as it sets the mood for my exercise sessions.

Investing in essential equipment was the next step in building my home gym. I carefully selected items that catered to my fitness goals and preferences. I began with an exercise mat, providing a comfortable surface for bodyweight exercises, yoga, and stretching. To incorporate strength training into my workouts, I purchased adjustable dumbbells and resistance bands. These versatile tools enable me to target various muscle groups effectively. Additionally, I added a stability ball to the mix for core workouts and balance exercises.

For cardiovascular workouts, I opted for a stationary exercise bike. It's a compact and user-friendly piece of equipment that allows me to elevate my heart rate, burn calories, and engage in low-impact cardio exercises right at home. While my choice was an exercise bike, others might prefer options like a treadmill, elliptical machine, or even a simple jump rope for cardio.

Creating an inspiring workout environment was vital for my motivation. I introduced a small sound system, helping me establish a motivating workout playlist that keeps me energized during sessions. Along with the music, I added motivational quotes and fitness posters to the walls of my home gym. These visual cues serve as reminders of my goals and inspire me to push through challenging workouts.

Organization and tidiness are essential in my home gym. I ensured that every piece of equipment had a designated storage space, keeping my workout area clutter-free and easily accessible. This organizational aspect has helped me transition seamlessly from one exercise to the next and minimize distractions, allowing me to focus entirely on my workouts.

Setting up my home gym has not only improved the convenience of my workouts but has also allowed me to create a personalized and inspiring space to pursue my fitness goals. It's an investment in my health and well-being that has made regular exercise more accessible and enjoyable.

safety precautions

Safety is of paramount importance when setting up and using a home gym. Neglecting safety precautions can lead to accidents and injuries that could disrupt your fitness journey. Here are some key safety precautions to consider when creating a home gym:

Space and Ventilation: Ensure your workout area has sufficient space for your equipment and movements. Adequate ventilation is crucial to prevent overheating and provide a comfortable exercise environment.

Lighting: Proper lighting is essential for safety. Well-lit spaces help you avoid tripping over equipment or losing balance during exercises. Invest in good-quality lighting to illuminate the area.

Equipment Placement: Arrange your equipment in a way that minimizes the risk of accidents. Keep items like weights and resistance bands organized and stored securely when not in use to prevent tripping hazards.

Flooring: Use appropriate flooring, such as rubber mats or interlocking tiles, to cushion your movements and reduce the impact on your joints. This also helps protect your floors from damage.

Equipment Maintenance: Regularly inspect and maintain your fitness equipment. Check for loose screws, frayed cables, or any signs of wear and tear. Faulty equipment can be dangerous, so address any issues promptly.

Warm-Up and Cool-Down: Always start your workout with a proper warm-up to prepare your muscles and joints for exercise. Likewise, conclude your workout with a cool-down and stretching routine to reduce the risk of injury.

Safety Equipment: If you're using heavy weights, a weightlifting belt may be necessary to protect your back during heavy lifting. Additionally, consider investing in weightlifting gloves to improve grip and protect your hands.

Supervision: If you have young children or pets in your home, make sure to exercise when they are not in the gym area or provide proper supervision to prevent accidents.

Emergency Plan: Keep a phone or an emergency contact nearby, and be prepared for any potential health issues. Having a first-aid kit available is also a wise precaution.

Proper Technique: Learn and practice proper exercise technique. Improper form is a common cause of injuries. Consider hiring a personal trainer or using online resources to ensure you're performing exercises correctly.

Hydration: Always have a water bottle nearby to stay hydrated during your workouts, especially during intense sessions.

Know Your Limits: Avoid pushing yourself too hard or lifting weights that are beyond your capacity. Gradually progress and challenge yourself safely.

Consult a Professional: If you have any underlying health conditions or are new to exercise, consult with a healthcare professional or fitness expert to create a safe and effective workout plan tailored to your needs.

By implementing these safety precautions, you can enjoy the benefits of a home gym without compromising your well-being. Safety should always be a top priority to ensure a sustainable and injury-free fitness journey.

Bodyweight Exercises
Push-ups

Push-ups are a versatile and effective exercise that target multiple muscle groups, primarily the chest, triceps, and shoulders. Here are step-by-step instructions on how to perform a standard push-up:

Starting Position:

Begin by finding a clear, flat surface, such as the floor or a yoga mat.

Position yourself face down on the floor with your hands placed slightly wider than shoulder-width apart.

Your toes should be touching the ground, and your body should form a straight line from your head to your heels. Engage your core muscles to maintain this alignment.

Execution:

Inhale and lower your body by bending your elbows. Keep your elbows close to your body at around a 45-degree angle from your torso. Your chest should come close to the ground, but do not let it touch.

Keep your back straight, and maintain a straight line from head to heels throughout the movement.

Exhale and push your body back up to the starting position, fully extending your arms. This completes one repetition.

Tips:

• Keep your core engaged throughout the exercise to maintain a straight line from head to heels.

• Focus on controlled movements and avoid rapid or jerky motions.

• Don't allow your hips to sag or rise; maintain a straight body position.

• Keep your neck in a neutral position by looking down at the floor a few feet in front of you.

• If you're a beginner, you can start with modified push-ups by keeping your knees on the ground while following the same form principles.

• As you progress, aim to increase the number of repetitions or try more challenging push-up variations, such as diamond push-ups, wide-grip push-ups, or decline push-ups.

Common Mistakes to Avoid:

Letting your lower back sag: Maintain a straight line from head to heels.

Allowing your elbows to flare out: Keep your elbows close to your body to protect your shoulders.

Only partial range of motion: Try to lower your chest close to the ground without touching it.

Rushing through the exercise: Focus on controlled, deliberate movements for maximum benefit.

Push-ups can be customized to suit your fitness level and goals. Whether you're a beginner or an advanced athlete, mastering proper push-up form is essential for building strength and endurance.

Pull-ups

Pull-ups are a challenging bodyweight exercise that primarily targets the muscles in your back, as well as your biceps, shoulders, and core. They are an excellent way to build upper body strength and improve your posture. Here's how to perform a pull-up with proper form:

1. Find a Sturdy Horizontal Bar:

- Locate a horizontal bar that can support your body weight.

2. Grip the Bar:

- Stand underneath the bar and reach up to grip it with your palms facing away from your body. Your hands should be slightly wider than shoulder-width apart.

3. Hang from the Bar:

- Hang from the bar with your arms fully extended and your body relaxed. Your legs should be straight, and your feet should not touch the ground.

4. Engage Your Core:

- Before you begin the pull-up, engage your core muscles to maintain proper body alignment throughout the exercise.

5. Start the Pull:

- Begin the pull-up by exhaling and pulling your chest toward the bar. Think about driving your elbows down and back while squeezing your shoulder blades together.

6. Chin Over the Bar:

• Continue pulling until your chin is over the bar or as close to it as you can get.

7. Lower Yourself Down:

• In a controlled manner, inhale and slowly lower your body back down to the starting position with your arms fully extended. Avoid swinging or dropping suddenly.

8. Repeat:

• Perform your desired number of repetitions.

Tips for Pull-Ups:

• If you're a beginner or working on building strength, you can use an assisted pull-up machine, resistance bands, or a spotter to help you perform the exercise.

• Maintain proper form throughout the exercise, keeping your body in a straight line from head to heels.

• Avoid using momentum or swinging to lift your body. This reduces the effectiveness of the exercise and increases the risk of injury.

• As you progress, you can try different grip variations, such as wide-grip pull-ups, close-grip pull-ups, or chin-ups, to target your muscles from various angles.

• Start with a manageable number of repetitions and gradually increase as you get stronger.

Pull-ups can be challenging, especially for beginners, but with consistent practice and dedication, you can build the necessary strength to perform this exercise effectively. They are an excellent addition to any fitness routine for developing upper body strength and enhancing your overall physical fitness.

Bodyweight Squats:

1. Stand with Proper Alignment: Begin by standing with your feet shoulder-width apart. Your toes should be slightly turned outwards, and your chest should be up with your shoulders relaxed.

2. Engage Your Core: Before you start the squat, engage your core muscles to stabilize your torso.

3. Initiate the Movement: Lower your body by bending your knees and pushing your hips back as if you were sitting in an imaginary chair. Keep your back straight, and don't round your shoulders.

4. Depth: Ideally, aim to squat until your thighs are parallel to the ground or as low as your mobility allows. Your knees should not go beyond your toes, and your weight should be on your heels.

5. Push Through Your Heels: Push through your heels and extend your hips and knees to return to the starting position. Keep your back straight throughout the movement.

6. Repeat: Perform your desired number of repetitions. A set of 10-20 squats is a good starting point, but adjust based on your fitness level.

Goblet Squats (with a Dumbbell or Kettlebell):

1. Hold a dumbbell or kettlebell close to your chest with both hands.

2. Perform the squat as described above, keeping the weight close to your body.

3. Goblet squats can be a great way to add resistance to your squats and increase the intensity of your workout.

Tips for Squats:

- Keep your chest up and your back straight to maintain proper form and reduce the risk of injury.

- Maintain a controlled pace, both on the way down and on the way up, to engage your muscles effectively.

- If you're new to squats, you can start with partial squats and gradually work towards deeper squats as your flexibility and strength improve.

- To make squats more challenging, you can try one-legged squats (pistol squats) or add weight by holding a dumbbell or kettlebell.

Squats are a versatile exercise that can be incorporated into your home workout routine to strengthen your lower body and improve your overall fitness. Remember to use proper form and start with a weight or depth that matches your current fitness level, then progress gradually as you get stronger.

Lunges:

1. Starting Position: Begin by standing with your feet hip-width apart and your hands on your hips.

2. Step Forward: Take a step forward with your right foot. The step should be long enough that when you lower your body, both knees form right angles, with your front knee positioned directly above your ankle.

3. Lower Your Body: Bend both knees to lower your body down towards the floor. Your back knee should come close to but not touch the ground.

4. Maintain Proper Alignment: Keep your torso upright, and ensure that your front knee doesn't extend beyond your toes. Your weight should be evenly distributed between both legs.

5. Push Back Up: Push through your front heel to return to the starting position.

6. Repeat on the Other Side: Alternate between your right and left legs for the desired number of repetitions. A set of 10-20 lunges on each leg is a good starting point.

Tips for Lunges:

- Engage your core muscles to maintain balance and stability.

- To add intensity, you can hold dumbbells in each hand, place your hands behind your head, or perform walking lunges by taking consecutive steps.

- Make sure your knee doesn't touch the ground forcefully; it should hover just above the floor to avoid unnecessary strain.

- Keep your movements controlled and maintain proper alignment throughout the exercise.

Lunges are an effective lower body workout that targets your quadriceps, hamstrings, and glutes. They are a versatile exercise that can be incorporated into your home workout routine to help improve lower body strength and overall fitness.

Planks:

1. Starting Position: Begin by lying face down on the floor or on an exercise mat. Place your elbows directly under your shoulders, so your forearms are flat on the ground. Your toes should be tucked under with your legs extended and your body in a straight line from head to heels.

2. Engage Your Core: Lift your body off the ground by pushing up onto your forearms and toes. Keep your body in a straight line, making sure your hips are neither too high nor sagging. Your core should be engaged, and your back should be flat.

3. Hold the Position: Maintain this position for as long as you can, ideally starting with 20-30 seconds for beginners and working your way up to longer durations as you build strength. Focus on your breath and stay as steady as possible.

4. Proper Alignment: Ensure that your neck is in line with your spine, and your gaze should be slightly in front of you. This helps maintain proper neck and spine alignment.

5. Breathe: Remember to breathe throughout the exercise. Don't hold your breath. Inhale and exhale slowly and steadily.

6. Exit the Plank: When you're ready to end the exercise, gently lower your body back to the floor.

Tips for Planks:

- Focus on maintaining a straight line from your head to your heels. Avoid letting your hips sag or hiking them up.

- Engage your core muscles throughout the exercise to stabilize your body.

- Start with shorter durations and gradually increase the time you can hold the plank as your core strength improves.

- You can perform planks in various ways, such as side planks, forearm planks, and high planks to target different areas of your core and upper body.

- Planks are a versatile exercise that can be included in your home workout routine to build core strength, improve posture, and enhance overall stability.

Planks are an effective isometric exercise for strengthening your core and stabilizing your entire body. They can be done at home with no equipment, making them a convenient and valuable addition to your fitness routine.

Burpee

A burpee is a full-body exercise that can be performed as part of a home workout to improve your cardiovascular fitness, build strength, and enhance endurance. Here's a simple burpee workout you can do at home:

Basic Burpee:

1. Stand with your feet shoulder-width apart.

2. Drop into a squat position, placing your hands on the floor in front of you.

3. Kick your feet back into a plank position.

4. Perform a push-up (optional).

5. Quickly jump your feet back to the squat position.

6. Explode up from the squat, jumping as high as you can.

7. Land softly and immediately go into the next repetition.

Home Burpee Workout:

1. Warm-up: Spend 5-10 minutes warming up with light cardio exercises like jumping jacks, jogging in place, or high knees.

2. Workout:

- Perform 3 sets of 10-15 burpees per set, with 30-60 seconds of rest between each set.

- You can adjust the number of burpees and rest intervals based on your fitness level. Beginners might start with fewer burpees and longer rest periods.

3. Cool-down: After completing the burpee sets, cool down with 5-10 minutes of stretching exercises. Focus on stretching your legs, back, and arms.

4. Hydration and Recovery: Make sure to stay hydrated throughout your workout and after. Replenish lost fluids and have a healthy post-workout snack or meal to aid in recovery.

Remember to maintain proper form during each burpee to prevent injury. If you're a beginner or have any health concerns, it's a good idea to consult with a fitness professional or your healthcare provider before starting any new exercise program. Additionally, you can modify the burpee by omitting the push-up or adjusting the intensity to suit your fitness level.

Mountain Climbers

Mountain climbers are a great bodyweight exercise that you can easily incorporate into your home workout routine. They work your core, legs, and provide a cardiovascular benefit. Here's how to do mountain climbers as part of a home workout:

:

1. Start in a high plank position with your hands directly under your shoulders and your body in a straight line from head to heels.

2. Engage your core and keep your back flat.

3. Begin by bringing your right knee toward your chest, keeping your toes off the ground.

4. Return your right leg to the plank position and immediately bring your left knee toward your chest.

5. Alternate between your right and left legs in a running or "climbing" motion.

1. **Warm-up: Spend 5-10 minutes warming up with light cardio exercises like jumping jacks, jogging in place, or high knees.**

2. **Workout:**

- **Perform 3 sets of mountain climbers, with each set lasting for 30 seconds to 1 minute, depending on your fitness level.**

- **Rest for 30-60 seconds between each set.**

3. **Cool-down: After completing the mountain climber sets, cool down with 5-10 minutes of stretching exercises, focusing on stretching your core, legs, and arms.**

4. Hydration and Recovery: Stay hydrated during your workout and after. Have a healthy post-workout snack or meal to support recovery.

If you're a beginner, you can start with shorter intervals and increase the duration as you become more comfortable with the exercise. Ensure you maintain good form, keeping your core engaged and your back straight. Mountain climbers are an effective exercise for building endurance and strength in your core and lower body.

If you're a beginner, you can start with shorter intervals and increase the duration as you become more comfortable with the exercise. Ensure you maintain good form, keeping your core engaged and your back straight. Mountain climbers are an effective exercise for building endurance and strength in your core and lower body.

Bicycle crunches

Bicycle crunches are a fantastic home workout exercise that targets your abdominal muscles and obliques. Here's how to perform bicycle crunches and incorporate them into your workout routine:

1. Start by lying on your back on a comfortable surface, such as a yoga mat or carpet.

2. Place your hands lightly behind your head, without pulling on your neck, to support your head and neck.

3. Lift your legs off the ground and bend your knees at a 90-degree angle. Your lower legs should be parallel to the floor.

4. Lift your shoulder blades off the ground to engage your core.

5. Bring your right elbow towards your left knee while extending your right leg straight out. Simultaneously, bring your left knee toward your chest.

6. Switch sides, bringing your left elbow towards your right knee while extending your left leg straight out.

7. Continue this pedaling motion, as if you're riding a bicycle, while engaging your core and twisting your torso.

Here's a simple home workout routine with bicycle crunches:

1. Warm-up: Begin with a 5-10 minute warm-up that includes light cardio exercises like jogging in place or jumping jacks.

2. Workout:

- Perform 3 sets of bicycle crunches.

- Aim for 12-15 repetitions per side in each set.

- Rest for 30-60 seconds between each set.

3. Cool-down: After completing the bicycle crunch sets, cool down with 5-10 minutes of stretching exercises, focusing on your core, legs, and arms.

4. Hydration and Recovery: Stay hydrated during your workout and after. Have a healthy post-workout snack or meal to support recovery.

As you get more comfortable with bicycle crunches, you can increase the number of repetitions or sets. Be mindful of your form and avoid pulling on your neck when placing your hands behind your head. Bicycle crunches are excellent for strengthening your abdominal muscles and improving your core stability.

High Knees

High knees are a dynamic and effective cardio exercise that can be included in your home workout routine. They help improve cardiovascular fitness, leg strength, and agility. Here's how to perform high knees and create a home workout using this exercise:

1. Stand with your feet hip-width apart and keep your arms by your sides.

2. Begin jogging in place, lifting your knees as high as possible with each step.

3. Engage your core and keep your back straight as you jog.

4. Pump your arms in sync with your legs for added intensity.

Here's a simple home workout routine with high knees:

1. Warm-up: Start with a 5-10 minute warm-up that includes light cardio exercises like jogging in place, jumping jacks, or dynamic stretches to loosen up your muscles.

2. Workout:

- Perform 3 sets of high knees.

- Aim for 30-60 seconds of high knees in each set.

- Rest for 30-60 seconds between each set.

3. Cool-down: After completing the high knees sets, cool down with 5-10 minutes of static stretching exercises, targeting your legs, hips, and arms.

4. Hydration and Recovery: Stay hydrated during your workout and after. Have a healthy post-workout snack or meal to support recovery.

For a more challenging workout, you can increase the duration of your high knees or incorporate high knees into a high-intensity interval training (HIIT) routine by alternating them with other exercises. The key is to maintain good form, keeping your knees high and moving at a brisk pace. High knees are an excellent way to elevate your heart rate and add an element of intensity to your home workouts.

High knees are a dynamic and effective cardio exercise that can be included in your home workout routine. They help improve cardiovascular fitness, leg strength, and agility. Here's how to perform high knees and create a home workout using this exercise:

High Knees:

1. Stand with your feet hip-width apart and keep your arms by your sides.

2. Begin jogging in place, lifting your knees as high as possible with each step.

3. Engage your core and keep your back straight as you jog.

4. Pump your arms in sync with your legs for added intensity.

For a more challenging workout, you can increase the duration of your high knees or incorporate high knees into a high-intensity interval training (HIIT) routine by alternating them with other exercises. The key is to maintain good form, keeping your knees high and moving at a brisk pace. High knees are an excellent way to elevate your heart rate and add an element of intensity to your home workouts.

Dumbbell Workouts
Dumbbell Rows:

Dumbbell rows are an excellent home workout exercise for targeting your back, particularly the latissimus dorsi muscles (lats). Here's how to perform dumbbell rows at home:

Dumbbell Rows:

Stand with your feet hip-width apart, holding a dumbbell in each hand by your sides.

Bend your knees slightly and hinge at your hips, keeping your back straight and your chest up. This is your starting position.

Engage your core and keep your back flat as you bend forward at your hips. Your upper body should be almost parallel to the ground.

Hold the dumbbells with your palms facing your body. Your arms should hang straight down from your shoulders.

To perform the row, pull the dumbbells up to your hips, keeping your elbows close to your body. Squeeze your shoulder blades together at the top of the movement.

Lower the dumbbells back down to the starting position in a controlled manner.

Here's a simple home workout routine using dumbbell rows:

Warm-up: Begin with a 5-10 minute warm-up that includes light cardio exercises, like jogging in place or jumping jacks, to get your heart rate up and prepare your muscles.

Workout:

- Perform 3 sets of dumbbell rows.

- Aim for 8-12 repetitions in each set. Choose a weight that challenges you but allows you to maintain proper form.

- Rest for 30-60 seconds between each set.

Cool-down: After completing the dumbbell row sets, cool down with 5-10 minutes of stretching exercises, focusing on your back, shoulders, and arms.

Hydration and Recovery: Stay hydrated during your workout and after. Have a healthy post-workout snack or meal to support recovery.

Dumbbell rows are an effective exercise for strengthening your back muscles and improving posture. Ensure that you maintain good form throughout the exercise, and be cautious not to use too much weight, which could compromise your form and increase the risk of injury.

Dumbbell bicep curls

Dumbbell bicep curls are a popular and effective home workout exercise for building and toning the biceps. Here's how to perform dumbbell bicep curls:

1. Stand with your feet hip-width apart and hold a dumbbell in each hand, with your arms fully extended and your palms facing forward. This is your starting position.

2. Keep your back straight, chest up, and core engaged.

3. Without moving your upper arms, slowly bend your elbows and curl the dumbbells toward your shoulders while exhaling. Keep your wrists straight during the movement.

4. Contract your biceps at the top of the movement, then lower the dumbbells back to the starting position in a controlled manner while inhaling.

5. Repeat for the desired number of repetitions.

Here's a simple home workout routine using dumbbell bicep curls:

Warm-up: Begin with a 5-10 minute warm-up that includes light cardio exercises and dynamic stretches to get your blood flowing and prepare your muscles.

Workout:

- Perform 3 sets of dumbbell bicep curls.

- Aim for 10-15 repetitions per set. Choose a weight that is challenging but allows you to maintain proper form.

- Rest for 30-60 seconds between each set.

Cool-down: After completing the dumbbell bicep curl sets, cool down with 5-10 minutes of static stretching exercises, focusing on your biceps, shoulders, and arms.

Hydration and Recovery: Stay hydrated during your workout and after. Have a healthy post-workout snack or meal to support recovery.

Dumbbell bicep curls are an excellent way to build strength and size in your biceps. Maintaining proper form and using controlled movements is essential to maximize the effectiveness of this exercise and minimize the risk of injury. Adjust the weight as needed to suit your fitness level and goals.

Dumbbell Tricep Extensions (Skull Crushers):

Dumbbell tricep extensions, also known as dumbbell skull crushers, are a great home workout exercise to target and strengthen the triceps. Here's how to perform dumbbell tricep extensions:

1. Lie on your back on a bench or a stable surface, such as the floor. Hold a dumbbell in each hand with your arms fully extended above your chest. Your palms should be facing each other.

2. Bend your elbows and lower the dumbbells towards your forehead, keeping your upper arms stationary. Your elbows should create a 90-degree angle.

3. Engage your triceps to extend your elbows and push the dumbbells back to the starting position.

4. Ensure a controlled and smooth motion throughout the exercise, avoiding any sudden or jerky movements.

Here's a simple home workout routine using dumbbell tricep extensions:

Warm-up: Start with a 5-10 minute warm-up that includes light cardio exercises and dynamic stretches to prepare your muscles.

Workout:

- Perform 3 sets of dumbbell tricep extensions.

- Aim for 10-15 repetitions per set. Choose a weight that challenges you but allows you to maintain proper form.

- Rest for 30-60 seconds between each set.

Cool-down: After completing the tricep extension sets, cool down with 5-10 minutes of static stretching exercises, focusing on your triceps, shoulders, and arms.

Hydration and Recovery: Stay hydrated during your workout and after. Have a healthy post-workout snack or meal to support recovery.

Dumbbell tricep extensions are a powerful exercise for building and toning the triceps, the muscles on the back of your upper arms. It's crucial to maintain good form to avoid unnecessary strain on the elbows and wrists. You can adjust the weight to match your fitness level and gradually increase it as you get stronger.

Dumbbell lunges

Dumbbell lunges are a challenging and effective lower body exercise that can be incorporated into your home workout routine to strengthen your legs, glutes, and core. Here's how to perform dumbbell lunges:

1. Starting Position: Begin by standing upright with a dumbbell in each hand. Let your arms hang naturally by your sides. Make sure you have enough space to step forward and backward.

2. Step Forward: Take a step forward with your right leg. The length of your step should be such that when you lower your body, both knees form right angles, with your front knee positioned directly above your ankle.

3. Lower Your Body: Bend both knees to lower your body down towards the floor. Your back knee should come close to but not touch the ground. Ensure that your front knee does not extend beyond your toes.

4. Maintain Proper Alignment: Keep your torso upright, and ensure that your front knee is aligned with your ankle and doesn't go beyond your toes. Your weight should be evenly distributed between both legs.

5. Push Back Up: Push through your front heel to return to the starting position.

6. Alternate Legs: After completing a lunge with one leg, alternate by stepping forward with your left leg for the next repetition.

7. Repeat: Continue to alternate between legs for the desired number of repetitions. A set of 10-20 lunges on each leg is a good starting point.

Tips for Dumbbell Lunges:

- Engage your core muscles to maintain balance and stability.

- Choose an appropriate weight for the dumbbells. They should be challenging but allow you to maintain proper form.

- Maintain a controlled pace and proper alignment throughout the exercise.

- To intensify the exercise, you can use heavier dumbbells or add a higher number of repetitions.

- Always start with a warm-up and perform stretches to improve your flexibility and prevent injuries.

Dumbbell lunges are an excellent addition to your home workout routine, targeting your lower body muscles effectively. They offer versatility and can be adjusted in terms of weight, repetitions, and variations to match your fitness level and goals.

Dumbbell Deadlifts:

Dumbbell deadlifts are an effective compound exercise that primarily targets the muscles of your lower back, glutes, hamstrings, and core. Here's how to perform dumbbell deadlifts in a home workout:

1. Stand with your feet hip-width apart, holding a dumbbell in each hand in front of your thighs. Your palms should face your body.

2. Keep your back straight, chest up, and core engaged.

3. Bend at your hips and knees, lowering the dumbbells towards the ground while keeping them close to your legs.

4. Lower the dumbbells until your back is almost parallel to the ground or as far as your flexibility allows. Your back should remain straight throughout the movement.

5. Push through your heels and stand back up, extending your hips and knees until you return to the starting position.

6. Keep the dumbbells close to your body as you lift them and lower them. Avoid rounding your back.

Here's a simple home workout routine using dumbbell deadlifts:

Warm-up: Begin with a 5-10 minute warm-up that includes light cardio exercises and dynamic stretches to prepare your muscles.

Workout:

- Perform 3 sets of dumbbell deadlifts.

- Aim for 8-12 repetitions per set. Choose a weight that is challenging but allows you to maintain proper form.

- Rest for 30-60 seconds between each set.

Cool-down: After completing the deadlift sets, cool down with 5-10 minutes of stretching exercises, focusing on your lower back, glutes, hamstrings, and legs.

Hydration and Recovery: Stay hydrated during your workout and after. Have a healthy post-workout snack or meal to support recovery.

Dumbbell deadlifts are an excellent exercise for building lower body strength and enhancing your overall stability. Proper form is crucial to avoid injury, so ensure that your back remains straight and your movements are controlled throughout the exercise. Adjust the weight as needed to match your fitness level and goals.

Dumbbell Squats:

Dumbbell squats are a great home workout exercise to strengthen your lower body, including your quadriceps, hamstrings, glutes, and even your core. Here's a step-by-step guide on how to perform dumbbell squats:

1. Start by standing with your feet shoulder-width apart, holding a dumbbell in each hand at your sides. Your palms should be facing inward, and the dumbbells should hang alongside your thighs.

2. Keep your back straight, chest up, and your core engaged. This will help maintain good posture and protect your lower back.

3. Begin the squat by simultaneously bending at your hips and knees, as if you're sitting back into an imaginary chair. Lower your body while keeping your back straight. Your knees should be in line with your toes.

4. Continue lowering yourself until your thighs are parallel to the ground, or go as far as your flexibility allows without compromising your form. It's important to maintain your balance throughout the movement.

5. Push through your heels to stand back up, extending your hips and knees. Return to the starting position.

6. Remember to keep the dumbbells close to your body throughout the exercise, and ensure your knees don't extend beyond your toes.

Here's a simple home workout routine using dumbbell squats:

Warm-up: Start with a 5-10 minute warm-up that includes light cardio exercises and dynamic stretches to prepare your muscles.

Workout:

- Perform 3 sets of dumbbell squats.

- Aim for 10-15 repetitions per set. Choose a weight that challenges you but allows you to maintain proper form.

- Rest for 30-60 seconds between each set.

Cool-down: After completing the squat sets, cool down with 5-10 minutes of stretching exercises, focusing on your quadriceps, hamstrings, glutes, and lower body.

Hydration and Recovery: Stay hydrated during your workout and after. Have a healthy post-workout snack or meal to support recovery.

Dumbbell squats are a versatile exercise for building lower body strength and stability. Proper form is crucial to avoid injury, so ensure your back stays straight and your movements are controlled throughout the exercise. You can adjust the weight to match your fitness level and gradually increase it as you get stronger.

Dumbbell Shoulder Press:

The dumbbell shoulder press is an effective exercise for strengthening the shoulder muscles, particularly the deltoids. Here's how to perform a dumbbell shoulder press as part of your home workout:

1. Sit on a bench with a backrest, or stand with your feet shoulder-width apart, depending on your preference and equipment available. If you're sitting, make sure the backrest is set at a 90-degree angle or close to it.

2. Hold a dumbbell in each hand at shoulder height with your palms facing forward and your elbows bent. Your upper arms should be parallel to the ground, forming a 90-degree angle with your forearms.

3. Engage your core to stabilize your spine and maintain good posture.

4. Press the dumbbells upward by extending your arms fully while exhaling. Keep your wrists straight throughout the movement.

5. At the top of the movement, your arms should be fully extended overhead.

6. Lower the dumbbells back down to shoulder height while inhaling. Ensure a controlled and smooth motion throughout the exercise.

Here's a simple home workout routine using dumbbell shoulder presses:

Warm-up: Begin with a 5-10 minute warm-up that includes light cardio exercises, such as jumping jacks, and dynamic stretches to prepare your shoulder joints and muscles.

Workout:

- Perform 3 sets of dumbbell shoulder presses.

- Aim for 8-12 repetitions per set. Choose a weight that challenges you but allows you to maintain proper form.

- Rest for 30-60 seconds between each set.

Cool-down: After completing the shoulder press sets, cool down with 5-10 minutes of stretching exercises, focusing on your shoulders, arms, and upper body.

Hydration and Recovery: Stay hydrated during your workout and after. Have a healthy post-workout snack or meal to support recovery.

Dumbbell shoulder presses are excellent for building shoulder strength and improving overall shoulder stability. Maintain proper form throughout the exercise to avoid unnecessary strain on your shoulders and neck. You can adjust the weight to match your fitness level and gradually increase it as you get stronger.

Dumbbell Russian Twists:

Dumbbell Russian twists are a core-strengthening exercise that also engages your oblique muscles. Here's how to perform dumbbell Russian twists as part of your home workout:

1. Sit on the floor with your knees bent and your feet flat. You can elevate your feet a few inches off the ground to make the exercise more challenging.

2. Hold a dumbbell with both hands, gripping it close to your chest.

3. Lean back slightly to engage your core muscles and maintain balance.

4. Lift your feet off the ground (if not already elevated) and cross your ankles, or keep them side by side.

5. Rotate your torso to the right, bringing the dumbbell toward the floor beside your hip.

6. Return to the center and then rotate your torso to the left, bringing the dumbbell toward the floor beside your opposite hip.

7. Continue this twisting motion, making sure to engage your core throughout the exercise.

8. Perform the desired number of repetitions on each side.

Here's a simple home workout routine using dumbbell Russian twists:

Warm-up: Begin with a 5-10 minute warm-up that includes light cardio exercises and dynamic stretches to prepare your core and other muscles.

Workout:
- Perform 3 sets of dumbbell Russian twists.
- Aim for 12-20 twists (6-10 twists per side) in each set.

- Rest for 30-60 seconds between each set.

Cool-down: After completing the Russian twist sets, cool down with 5-10 minutes of stretching exercises, focusing on your core, obliques, and lower back.

Hydration and Recovery: Stay hydrated during your workout and after. Have a healthy post-workout snack or meal to support recovery.

Dumbbell Russian twists are a great exercise for working your core and oblique muscles. Maintaining proper form and engaging your core muscles is essential to maximize the effectiveness of this exercise and minimize the risk of injury. You can adjust the weight of the dumbbell and the number of repetitions to match your fitness level and goals.

Dumbbell Farmer's Walk:

Dumbbell Farmer's Walk is an effective full-body exercise that helps improve grip strength, core stability, and overall muscle endurance. It's a simple but highly functional movement that simulates carrying heavy objects. Here's how to perform the Dumbbell Farmer's Walk as part of your home workout:

1. Select two dumbbells of appropriate weight for your fitness level. The weight should be challenging but manageable.

2. Stand with your feet shoulder-width apart and place a dumbbell beside each foot.

3. Bend at the hips and knees to lower yourself, keeping your back straight. Reach down and grab the dumbbells with a firm grip.

4. Lift the dumbbells off the ground while maintaining a neutral spine and keeping your chest up.

5. Stand up straight, holding the dumbbells by your sides with your arms fully extended. Your shoulders should be down and back, and your core engaged.

6. Walk forward in a controlled manner, taking short, brisk steps. Keep your posture upright and your shoulders back.

7. Walk for a specific distance or time, depending on your fitness level and available space.

8. After completing the desired distance or time, lower the dumbbells back to the ground with proper form.

Here's a simple home workout routine using Dumbbell Farmer's Walk:

Warm-up: Start with a 5-10 minute warm-up that includes light cardio exercises and dynamic stretches to prepare your muscles.

Workout:

- Perform 3 sets of Dumbbell Farmer's Walks.

- Walk for a specific distance (e.g., 50-100 feet) or a certain duration (e.g., 30-60 seconds) in each set.

- Rest for 30-60 seconds between each set.

Cool-down: After completing the Farmer's Walk sets, cool down with 5-10 minutes of stretching exercises, focusing on your grip, legs, and core.

Hydration and Recovery: Stay hydrated during your workout and after. Have a healthy post-workout snack or meal to support recovery.

The Dumbbell Farmer's Walk is a functional exercise that not only strengthens your muscles but also enhances grip strength and core stability. Proper form is crucial to maximize its benefits and minimize the risk of injury. You can adjust the weight of the dumbbells and the distance or duration of the walk to match your fitness level and goals.

Dumbbell Bench Press:

The dumbbell bench press is a classic and effective upper body exercise that primarily targets the chest muscles but also engages the shoulders and triceps. Here's how to perform the dumbbell bench press as part of your home workout:

1. Lie on a bench with your back flat against the surface and your feet flat on the ground. Your knees should be bent at a 90-degree angle. If you don't have a bench, you can also do this exercise on the floor.

2. Hold a dumbbell in each hand with your arms extended and your palms facing forward. Your hands should be at chest level, and your elbows should be bent at a 90-degree angle. This is your starting position.

3. Lower the dumbbells to the sides of your chest, allowing your elbows to bend and your upper arms to come close to or just below parallel with the ground. Keep your wrists straight.

4. Push the dumbbells back up to the starting position while exhaling, extending your arms fully without locking your elbows.

5. Maintain a controlled and smooth motion throughout the exercise.

Here's a simple home workout routine using the dumbbell bench press:

Warm-up: Begin with a 5-10 minute warm-up that includes light cardio exercises and dynamic stretches to prepare your chest, shoulders, and arms.

Workout:

- Perform 3 sets of dumbbell bench presses.

- Aim for 8-12 repetitions per set. Choose a weight that challenges you but allows you to maintain proper form.

- Rest for 30-60 seconds between each set.

Cool-down: After completing the bench press sets, cool down with 5-10 minutes of stretching exercises, focusing on your chest, shoulders, and arms.

Hydration and Recovery: Stay hydrated during your workout and after. Have a healthy post-workout snack or meal to support recovery.

The dumbbell bench press is an effective exercise for building chest strength and overall upper body stability. Proper form is essential to avoid injury, so make sure you maintain a stable and controlled motion throughout the exercise. You can adjust the weight to match your fitness level and gradually increase it as you get stronger.

Kettlebell Workouts

Kettlebell Swings:

Kettlebell swings are a dynamic and effective full-body exercise that primarily targets the posterior chain muscles, including the glutes, hamstrings, lower back, and core. Here's how to perform kettlebell swings as part of your home workout:

1. Stand with your feet shoulder-width apart, with a kettlebell on the floor in front of you.

2. Bend at the hips and knees to reach down and grab the kettlebell handle with both hands. Keep your back straight, chest up, and core engaged.

3. Swing the kettlebell backward between your legs while maintaining a slight bend in your knees. Hinge at your hips, keeping your back straight.

4. In one fluid motion, drive your hips forward and swing the kettlebell out in front of you. Your arms should remain straight, and the power should come from your hips and glutes.

5. As the kettlebell reaches shoulder height, your body should form a straight line from your head to your heels.

6. Let the kettlebell swing back between your legs, and immediately initiate the next swing by driving your hips forward.

7. Continue the swinging motion for the desired number of repetitions.

Here's a simple home workout routine using kettlebell swings:

Warm-up: Begin with a 5-10 minute warm-up that includes light cardio exercises and dynamic stretches to prepare your muscles and joints.

Workout:

- Perform 3 sets of kettlebell swings.
- Aim for 12-15 repetitions per set.
- Rest for 30-60 seconds between each set.

Cool-down: After completing the kettlebell swing sets, cool down with 5-10 minutes of stretching exercises, focusing on your hips, hamstrings, lower back, and core.

Hydration and Recovery: Stay hydrated during your workout and after. Have a healthy post-workout snack or meal to support recovery.

Kettlebell swings are a powerful exercise for improving your posterior chain strength and overall athletic performance. Proper form and a controlled swinging motion are essential to maximize the exercise's benefits and prevent injury. You can adjust the weight of the kettlebell to match your fitness level and gradually increase it as you get stronger.

Kettlebell Goblet Squats:

Kettlebell goblet squats are an effective lower body exercise that not only target the quadriceps, hamstrings, and glutes but also engage the core and upper body muscles. Here's how to perform kettlebell goblet squats as part of your home workout:

1. Stand with your feet shoulder-width apart, holding a kettlebell with both hands close to your chest. Hold the kettlebell handle with your palms facing upward.

2. Keep your back straight, chest up, and your core engaged. This is your starting position.

3. Initiate the squat by bending at your hips and knees, lowering your body as if you're sitting back into an imaginary chair. Keep your back straight, and your knees should be in line with your toes.

4. Continue lowering yourself until your thighs are parallel to the ground or as far as your flexibility allows.

5. Push through your heels to stand back up, extending your hips and knees until you return to the starting position.

6. Maintain the kettlebell close to your chest throughout the exercise, and keep your elbows pointing down.

Here's a simple home workout routine using kettlebell goblet squats:

Warm-up: Begin with a 5-10 minute warm-up that includes light cardio exercises and dynamic stretches to prepare your muscles.

Workout:

- Perform 3 sets of kettlebell goblet squats.

- Aim for 10-12 repetitions per set. Choose a kettlebell weight that challenges you but allows you to maintain proper form.

- Rest for 30-60 seconds between each set.

Cool-down: After completing the goblet squat sets, cool down with 5-10 minutes of stretching exercises, focusing on your legs, hips, and lower back.

Hydration and Recovery: Stay hydrated during your workout and after. Have a healthy post-workout snack or meal to support recovery.

Kettlebell goblet squats are a versatile exercise for building lower body strength and improving overall stability. Proper form is essential to avoid injury, so ensure that your back remains straight and your movements are controlled throughout the exercise. You can adjust the weight of the kettlebell to match your fitness level and gradually increase it as you get stronger.

Kettlebell Turkish Get-Ups:

Kettlebell Turkish get-ups are a challenging and comprehensive exercise that works multiple muscle groups while also enhancing stability and coordination. Here's how to perform kettlebell Turkish get-ups as part of your home workout:

1. Start by lying on your back on the floor with your legs straight and a kettlebell in one hand, arm extended toward the ceiling. Bend your knee on the same side as the kettlebell.

2. The opposite arm and leg should be extended straight out to your sides.

3. Begin the movement by rolling onto your side while maintaining a firm grip on the kettlebell.

4. Use your free hand to push off the ground, lifting your torso and straightening your supporting arm.

5. Lift your hips off the ground, creating a tripod-like position with your supporting arm, leg, and kettlebell arm.

6. Sweep your extended leg under your body and place it behind your knee as you come to a kneeling position.

7. Stand up from the kneeling position with the kettlebell extended overhead.

8. To return to the starting position, reverse the movement: step back into a kneeling position, sweep the leg back to a straight position, and lower your hips to the ground, followed by your back, while maintaining control of the kettlebell.

9. Repeat for the desired number of repetitions, then switch to the other arm.

Here's a simple home workout routine using kettlebell Turkish get-ups:

Warm-up: Begin with a 5-10 minute warm-up that includes light cardio exercises and dynamic stretches to prepare your muscles and joints.

Workout:

- Perform 3-4 sets of kettlebell Turkish get-ups per arm.

- Aim for 3-5 repetitions per set, focusing on quality and control.

- Rest for 60-90 seconds between sets.

Cool-down: After completing the Turkish get-ups, cool down with 5-10 minutes of stretching exercises, focusing on your shoulders, hips, and core.

Hydration and Recovery: Stay hydrated during your workout and after. Have a healthy post-workout snack or meal to support recovery.

Kettlebell Turkish get-ups are a complex exercise that demands proper form and controlled movements to avoid injury. They are highly effective for strengthening your core, shoulders, hips, and overall stability. You can adjust the weight of the kettlebell and the number of repetitions to match your fitness level and gradually increase the challenge as you get stronger.

Kettlebell Lunges:

Kettlebell lunges are a fantastic lower body exercise that targets your quadriceps, hamstrings, glutes, and calves. They also engage your core for stability. Here's how to perform kettlebell lunges as part of your home workout:

1. Start by standing upright with your feet together and holding a kettlebell in each hand at your sides. Keep your palms facing inwards.

2. Keep your back straight, chest up, and your core engaged.

3. Take a step forward with one leg while maintaining good posture. This will be your starting position.

4. Lower your body by bending both knees, ensuring your front knee doesn't extend past your toes, and your back knee hovers just above the ground.

5. Push through the heel of your front foot to stand back up, returning to the starting position.

6. Repeat the lunge with the opposite leg.

7. Continue alternating legs for the desired number of repetitions.

Here's a simple home workout routine using kettlebell lunges:

Warm-up: Start with a 5-10 minute warm-up that includes light cardio exercises and dynamic stretches to prepare your leg muscles and joints.

Workout:

- Perform 3 sets of kettlebell lunges.

- Aim for 10-12 lunges per leg in each set. Choose a kettlebell weight that challenges you but allows you to maintain proper form.

- Rest for 30-60 seconds between each set.

Cool-down: After completing the lunge sets, cool down with 5-10 minutes of stretching exercises, focusing on your legs, hips, and lower back.

Hydration and Recovery: Stay hydrated during your workout and after. Have a healthy post-workout snack or meal to support recovery.

Kettlebell lunges are an excellent exercise for building lower body strength and stability. Proper form is crucial to avoid injury, so ensure that your back remains straight, and your movements are controlled throughout the exercise. You can adjust the weight of the kettlebell and the number of repetitions to match your fitness level and gradually increase the challenge as you get stronger.

Kettlebell Rows:

Kettlebell rows are a compound exercise that primarily targets your back muscles, particularly the latissimus dorsi, while also engaging your biceps and shoulders. Here's how to perform kettlebell rows as part of your home workout:

1. Stand with your feet hip-width apart, holding a kettlebell in your right hand.

2. Bend your knees slightly and hinge at your hips to lean forward, keeping your back straight and your chest up. Your torso should be close to parallel to the ground.

3. Your left hand can rest on your left thigh or knee for support.

4. Hold the kettlebell in your right hand with your arm fully extended toward the ground.

5. Initiate the row by bending your right elbow, pulling the kettlebell toward your hip while keeping your upper arm close to your body.

6. Squeeze your shoulder blades together at the top of the movement to engage your back muscles.

7. Lower the kettlebell back down to the starting position with control.

8. Repeat for the desired number of repetitions on the right side, then switch to the left hand.

Here's a simple home workout routine using kettlebell rows:

Warm-up: Start with a 5-10 minute warm-up that includes light cardio exercises and dynamic stretches to prepare your muscles and joints.

Workout:

- Perform 3 sets of kettlebell rows for each arm.

- Aim for 8-12 repetitions per set. Choose a kettlebell weight that challenges you but allows you to maintain proper form.

- Rest for 30-60 seconds between each set.

Cool-down: After completing the kettlebell row sets, cool down with 5-10 minutes of stretching exercises, focusing on your back, shoulders, and arms.

Hydration and Recovery: Stay hydrated during your workout and after. Have a healthy post-workout snack or meal to support recovery.

Kettlebell rows are an effective exercise for strengthening your back muscles and improving posture. Proper form is crucial to avoid injury, so ensure that your back remains straight and your movements are controlled throughout the exercise. You can adjust the weight of the kettlebell to match your fitness level and gradually increase it as you get stronger.

Kettlebell Snatches:

Kettlebell snatches are a dynamic full-body exercise that engages multiple muscle groups and improves strength, power, and cardiovascular fitness. Here's how to perform kettlebell snatches as part of your home workout:

1. Start by placing a kettlebell on the ground in front of you.

2. Stand with your feet shoulder-width apart and hinge at your hips and knees to lower yourself into a squat position.

3. Reach down and grasp the kettlebell with one hand, keeping your palm facing your body.

4. Swing the kettlebell between your legs while maintaining a straight back and engaged core.

5. As the kettlebell swings back, forcefully extend your hips and knees to generate momentum. When the kettlebell is at its highest point between your legs, use your hips to push it upward.

6. Simultaneously, pull the kettlebell up with your arm, bending your elbow to guide it to the overhead position.

7. In one fluid motion, fully extend your hips and knees, and lock out your arm with the kettlebell overhead.

8. Lower the kettlebell back down in a controlled manner, bending at the hips and knees while keeping your arm extended.

9. Swing the kettlebell back between your legs and repeat the motion for the desired number of repetitions.

10. Once you've completed the reps with one hand, switch to the other hand.

Here's a simple home workout routine using kettlebell snatches:

Warm-up: Begin with a 5-10 minute warm-up that includes light cardio exercises and dynamic stretches to prepare your muscles and joints.

Workout:

- Perform 3-4 sets of kettlebell snatches for each hand.

- Aim for 8-10 repetitions per set.

- Rest for 60-90 seconds between sets.

Cool-down: After completing the kettlebell snatch sets, cool down with 5-10 minutes of stretching exercises, focusing on your shoulders, hips, and core.

Hydration and Recovery: Stay hydrated during your workout and after. Have a healthy post-workout snack or meal to support recovery.

Kettlebell snatches are a highly effective exercise for building power, strength, and coordination. Proper form and a controlled swinging motion are essential to maximize the exercise's benefits and minimize the risk of injury. You can adjust the weight of the kettlebell and the number of repetitions to match your fitness level and gradually increase the challenge as you get stronger.

Kettlebell Deadlifts:

Kettlebell deadlifts are a fundamental exercise for strengthening the posterior chain, including the lower back, glutes, and hamstrings. Here's how to perform kettlebell deadlifts as part of your home workout:

1. Start by placing a kettlebell on the ground in front of you.

2. Stand with your feet shoulder-width apart, with your toes pointing slightly outward.

3. Bend at your hips and knees to lower yourself into a squat position, keeping your back straight and your chest up.

4. Reach down and grasp the kettlebell handle with both hands, keeping your palms facing your body. Your hands should be shoulder-width apart or slightly wider.

5. Engage your core, and ensure your back remains straight as you prepare to lift the kettlebell.

6. Push through your heels and stand up, extending your hips and knees simultaneously.

7. As you lift the kettlebell, keep it close to your body and maintain a neutral spine. Your back should remain straight throughout the movement.

8. Stand up fully with the kettlebell, extending your hips and knees, and your body should be in an upright position.

9. Reverse the movement by hinging at your hips and bending your knees to lower the kettlebell back to the ground. Keep your back straight as you lower it.

10. Complete the desired number of repetitions, maintaining proper form throughout the exercise.

Here's a simple home workout routine using kettlebell deadlifts:

Warm-up: Begin with a 5-10 minute warm-up that includes light cardio exercises and dynamic stretches to prepare your muscles and joints.

Workout:

- Perform 3-4 sets of kettlebell deadlifts.

- Aim for 8-12 repetitions per set.

- Rest for 60-90 seconds between sets.

Cool-down: After completing the deadlift sets, cool down with 5-10 minutes of stretching exercises, focusing on your lower back, glutes, and hamstrings.

Hydration and Recovery: Stay hydrated during your workout and after. Have a healthy post-workout snack or meal to support recovery.

Kettlebell deadlifts are an excellent exercise for building lower body strength and improving overall stability. Proper form is crucial to avoid injury, so ensure that your back remains straight and your movements are controlled throughout the exercise. You can adjust the weight of the kettlebell to match your fitness level and gradually increase it as you get stronger.

Kettlebell Halos:

Kettlebell halos are a unique and effective exercise for building shoulder stability and mobility. They also engage the core and upper body muscles. Here's how to perform kettlebell halos as part of your home workout:

1. Begin by standing with your feet shoulder-width apart.

2. Hold the kettlebell by the handle with both hands, gripping it with your palms facing upward. Your arms should be fully extended in front of you.

3. Keep your core engaged and maintain good posture throughout the exercise.

4. Start by moving the kettlebell around your head in a circular motion, as if you're drawing a halo or crown around your head.

5. As you move the kettlebell to the back of your head, let it pass behind your neck, then continue the circular motion to the front. Make sure the kettlebell remains close to your head and doesn't stray too far from it.

6. Perform the desired number of reps in one direction (e.g., clockwise), then reverse the direction for the same number of reps (e.g., counterclockwise).

Here's a simple home workout routine using kettlebell halos:

Warm-up: Begin with a 5-10 minute warm-up that includes light cardio exercises and dynamic stretches to prepare your shoulder and core muscles.

Workout:

- Perform 2-3 sets of kettlebell halos.

- Aim for 6-8 repetitions in each direction per set.

- Rest for 30-60 seconds between sets.

Cool-down: After completing the halos sets, cool down with 5-10 minutes of stretching exercises, focusing on your shoulders, neck, and upper body.

Hydration and Recovery: Stay hydrated during your workout and after. Have a healthy post-workout snack or meal to support recovery.

Kettlebell halos are an excellent exercise for shoulder mobility and stability, as well as core engagement. Proper form and control of the kettlebell throughout the circular motion are essential. You can adjust the weight of the kettlebell to match your fitness level and gradually increase it as you become more comfortable with the exercise.

Kettlebell Windmills:

Kettlebell windmills are an effective exercise for improving core strength, shoulder mobility, and flexibility in your hamstrings and hips. Here's how to perform kettlebell windmills as part of your home workout:

1. Start by standing with your feet slightly wider than shoulder-width apart.

2. Hold a kettlebell in one hand with your arm fully extended overhead, and your palm facing forward. Your other arm can be extended to your side for balance.

3. Keep your feet pointed forward, and your toes on the same side as the kettlebell foot should be slightly turned outward (about 45 degrees).

4. Begin by hinging at your hips, lowering your upper body to the side opposite to the hand with the kettlebell. Keep your back straight and your eyes on the kettlebell.

5. As you lower your body, maintain your arm's extension, and keep the kettlebell directly above your shoulder. Your free hand can slide down your opposite leg for support.

6. Lower your body as far as your flexibility allows while maintaining proper form, and keep the kettlebell over your shoulder.

7. Reverse the motion by pushing through your heel to stand back up, returning to the starting position.

8. Complete the desired number of repetitions on one side, then switch to the other hand and repeat the exercise.

Here's a simple home workout routine using kettlebell windmills:

Warm-up: Begin with a 5-10 minute warm-up that includes light cardio exercises and dynamic stretches to prepare your muscles and improve your flexibility.

Workout:

- Perform 3 sets of kettlebell windmills for each side.

- Aim for 6-8 repetitions per set on each side.

- Rest for 30-60 seconds between each set.

Cool-down: After completing the windmill sets, cool down with 5-10 minutes of stretching exercises, focusing on your hamstrings, hips, and shoulders.

Hydration and Recovery: Stay hydrated during your workout and after. Have a healthy post-workout snack or meal to support recovery.

Kettlebell windmills are a beneficial exercise for improving mobility, flexibility, and core strength. Proper form and control are essential to maximize the exercise's benefits and minimize the risk of injury. You can adjust the weight of the kettlebell to match your fitness level and gradually increase it as you get more comfortable with the exercise.

Kettlebell Windmills:

Kettlebell windmills are an effective exercise for improving core strength, shoulder mobility, and flexibility in your hamstrings and hips. Here's how to perform kettlebell windmills as part of your home workout:

1. Start by standing with your feet slightly wider than shoulder-width apart.

2. Hold a kettlebell in one hand with your arm fully extended overhead, and your palm facing forward. Your other arm can be extended to your side for balance.

3. Keep your feet pointed forward, and your toes on the same side as the kettlebell foot should be slightly turned outward (about 45 degrees).

4. Begin by hinging at your hips, lowering your upper body to the side opposite to the hand with the kettlebell. Keep your back straight and your eyes on the kettlebell.

5. As you lower your body, maintain your arm's extension, and keep the kettlebell directly above your shoulder. Your free hand can slide down your opposite leg for support.

6. Lower your body as far as your flexibility allows while maintaining proper form, and keep the kettlebell over your shoulder.

7. Reverse the motion by pushing through your heel to stand back up, returning to the starting position.

8. Complete the desired number of repetitions on one side, then switch to the other hand and repeat the exercise.

Here's a simple home workout routine using kettlebell windmills:

Warm-up: Begin with a 5-10 minute warm-up that includes light cardio exercises and dynamic stretches to prepare your muscles and improve your flexibility.

Workout:

- Perform 3 sets of kettlebell windmills for each side.

- Aim for 6-8 repetitions per set on each side.

- Rest for 30-60 seconds between each set.

Cool-down: After completing the windmill sets, cool down with 5-10 minutes of stretching exercises, focusing on your hamstrings, hips, and shoulders.

Hydration and Recovery: Stay hydrated during your workout and after. Have a healthy post-workout snack or meal to support recovery.

Kettlebell windmills are a beneficial exercise for improving mobility, flexibility, and core strength. Proper form and control are essential to maximize the exercise's benefits and minimize the risk of injury. You can adjust the weight of the kettlebell to match your fitness level and gradually increase it as you get more comfortable with the exercise.

Resistance Band Exercises
Resistance Band Chest Flyes:

Resistance band chest flyes are a great home workout exercise for targeting the pectoral muscles (chest) and the anterior deltoids (front of the shoulders). Here's how to perform resistance band chest flyes:

Attach your resistance band to a secure anchor point, such as a doorknob or a wall anchor, at chest height.

Stand with your back to the anchor point, holding one end of the resistance band in each hand.

Take a step forward with one foot, maintaining a staggered stance. This will create tension in the resistance band.

Begin with your arms extended in front of you at chest height, with a slight bend in your elbows. Your palms should be facing each other, and your hands should be slightly wider than shoulder-width apart.

Keep your core engaged and maintain good posture with a slight bend in your knees.

Start by opening your arms in a wide arc, squeezing your chest muscles as you pull your hands apart.

As your hands reach shoulder level, pause briefly to feel the contraction in your chest.

Slowly reverse the motion and bring your hands back to the starting position in front of your chest.

Perform the desired number of repetitions, focusing on a controlled and smooth motion.

Here's a simple home workout routine using resistance band chest flyes:

Warm-up: Begin with a 5-10 minute warm-up that includes light cardio exercises and dynamic stretches to prepare your chest and shoulder muscles.

Workout:

- Perform 3 sets of resistance band chest flyes.
- Aim for 12-15 repetitions per set.
- Rest for 30-60 seconds between each set.

Cool-down: After completing the chest flye sets, cool down with 5-10 minutes of stretching exercises, focusing on your chest and shoulders.

Hydration and Recovery: Stay hydrated during your workout and after. Have a healthy post-workout snack or meal to support recovery.

Resistance band chest flyes are an effective exercise for targeting your chest muscles and enhancing shoulder mobility. Proper form and control of the resistance band are essential to maximize the benefits of this exercise and reduce the risk of injury. You can adjust the resistance level of the band to match your fitness level and gradually increase it as you get stronger.

Resistance Band Rows:

Resistance band rows are a versatile and effective home workout exercise that primarily targets the upper back muscles, including the latissimus dorsi and the rhomboids, as well as the biceps. Here's how to perform resistance band rows:

1. Attach your resistance band to a secure anchor point at about waist height. You can use a door anchor, a sturdy pole, or any stable structure.

2. Stand facing the anchor point and hold the handles or grips of the resistance band in each hand. Your arms should be fully extended, and your palms should be facing each other.

3. Take a step back to create tension in the resistance band, ensuring your feet are shoulder-width apart.

4. Keep your core engaged and maintain good posture with a slight bend in your knees.

5. Start the rowing motion by pulling the handles toward your lower ribcage. Keep your elbows close to your body as you pull.

6. Squeeze your shoulder blades together at the end of the motion to engage the upper back muscles.

7. Slowly extend your arms back to the starting position in a controlled manner.

8. Perform the desired number of repetitions, focusing on a smooth and controlled motion.

Here's a simple home workout routine using resistance band rows:

Warm-up: Begin with a 5-10 minute warm-up that includes light cardio exercises and dynamic stretches to prepare your back and arms.

Workout:

- Perform 3 sets of resistance band rows.
- Aim for 12-15 repetitions per set.

- Rest for 30-60 seconds between each set.

Cool-down: After completing the rows sets, cool down with 5-10 minutes of stretching exercises, focusing on your back and arms.

Hydration and Recovery: Stay hydrated during your workout and after. Have a healthy post-workout snack or meal to support recovery.

Resistance band rows are a valuable exercise for strengthening your upper back and improving posture. Proper form and control of the resistance band are essential to maximize the exercise's benefits and minimize the risk of injury. You can adjust the resistance level of the band to match your fitness level and gradually increase it as you get stronger.

Resistance Band Tricep Extensions:

Resistance band tricep extensions are a fantastic home workout exercise for targeting the triceps, which are the muscles on the back of your upper arms. Here's how to perform resistance band tricep extensions:

1. Begin by attaching your resistance band to a secure anchor point above your head, such as a sturdy doorframe or a pull-up bar.

2. Stand facing away from the anchor point and hold the handle or grip of the resistance band in both hands, fully extended above your head.

3. Take a step forward to create tension in the resistance band, ensuring your feet are hip-width apart.

4. Keep your core engaged and maintain good posture with a slight bend in your knees.

5. Initiate the tricep extension by bending your elbows and lowering your hands behind your head. Your upper arms should remain close to your ears.

6. Extend your arms fully to push the resistance band back up to the starting position.

7. Squeeze your triceps at the end of the extension to engage them fully.

8. Perform the desired number of repetitions, focusing on a smooth and controlled motion.

Here's a simple home workout routine using resistance band tricep extensions:

Warm-up: Begin with a 5-10 minute warm-up that includes light cardio exercises and dynamic stretches to prepare your arms and shoulders.

Workout:

- Perform 3 sets of resistance band tricep extensions.
- Aim for 12-15 repetitions per set.
- Rest for 30-60 seconds between each set.

Cool-down: After completing the tricep extension sets, cool down with 5-10 minutes of stretching exercises, focusing on your triceps and arms.

Hydration and Recovery: Stay hydrated during your workout and after. Have a healthy post-workout snack or meal to support recovery.

Resistance band tricep extensions are an excellent exercise for building tricep strength and toning the back of your arms. Proper form and control of the resistance band are essential to maximize the exercise's benefits and reduce the risk of injury. You can adjust the resistance level of the band to match your fitness level and gradually increase it as you get stronger.

Resistance Band Leg Raises:

Resistance band leg raises are a great home workout exercise for targeting your leg muscles, particularly the quadriceps (front of the thighs) and hip flexors. Here's how to perform resistance band leg raises:

1. Attach your resistance band to a secure anchor point, such as a sturdy pole or a door anchor, near floor level.

2. Place the band around your ankles or feet, depending on the length and type of your resistance band. Situate yourself facing away from the anchor point.

3. Lie flat on your back on the floor with your legs straight and your arms at your sides.

4. Keep your hands under your hips or beneath your lower back to support your lower spine and reduce discomfort.

5. Engage your core by pressing your lower back into the floor.

6. Lift your legs off the ground by flexing your hip and raising them upward. Keep your legs as straight as possible.

7. Slowly lower your legs back to the starting position, maintaining control throughout the movement.

8. Perform the desired number of repetitions, focusing on a smooth and controlled motion.

Here's a simple home workout routine using resistance band leg raises:

Warm-up: Begin with a 5-10 minute warm-up that includes light cardio exercises and dynamic stretches to prepare your leg muscles and joints.

Workout:

- Perform 3 sets of resistance band leg raises.

- Aim for 12-15 repetitions per set.

- Rest for 30-60 seconds between each set.

Cool-down: After completing the leg raise sets, cool down with 5-10 minutes of stretching exercises, focusing on your legs and hip flexors.

Hydration and Recovery: Stay hydrated during your workout and after. Have a healthy post-workout snack or meal to support recovery.

Resistance band leg raises are a beneficial exercise for building leg strength and hip flexibility. Proper form and control of the resistance band are essential to maximize the exercise's benefits and reduce the risk of injury. You can adjust the resistance level of the band to match your fitness level and gradually increase it as you get stronger.

Resistance Band Glute Bridges:

Resistance band glute bridges are a home workout exercise that targets the gluteal muscles, specifically the gluteus maximus. Here's how to perform resistance band glute bridges:

1. Begin by placing a resistance band just above your knees and lying on your back on an exercise mat or the floor.

2. Bend your knees and place your feet flat on the ground, hip-width apart. Your arms should be resting by your sides with your palms facing down.

3. Engage your core and press your lower back into the ground to maintain a neutral spine.

4. Press your knees out against the resistance band to create tension in the band.

5. Lift your hips off the ground by pushing through your heels. As you lift, squeeze your glutes to raise your hips as high as you can.

6. At the top of the movement, your body should form a straight line from your shoulders to your knees.

7. Hold the bridge position for a moment, ensuring that you're still pressing out against the resistance band.

8. Lower your hips back down to the ground in a controlled manner, but don't let them rest on the floor between repetitions.

9. Perform the desired number of repetitions, keeping the resistance band engaged throughout the exercise.

Here's a simple home workout routine using resistance band glute bridges:

Warm-up: Begin with a 5-10 minute warm-up that includes light cardio exercises and dynamic stretches to prepare your glutes and hip muscles.

Workout:

- Perform 3 sets of resistance band glute bridges.
- Aim for 12-15 repetitions per set.
- Rest for 30-60 seconds between each set.

Cool-down: After completing the glute bridge sets, cool down with 5-10 minutes of stretching exercises, focusing on your hip and glute muscles.

Hydration and Recovery: Stay hydrated during your workout and after. Have a healthy post-workout snack or meal to support recovery.

Resistance band glute bridges are an excellent exercise for strengthening and toning your gluteal muscles. Proper form and control of the resistance band are essential to maximize the exercise's benefits and reduce the risk of injury. You can adjust the resistance level of the band to match your fitness level and gradually increase it as you get stronger.

Resistance Band Side Leg Raises:

Resistance band side leg raises are a home workout exercise that targets the hip abductors, specifically the muscles on the outer thighs. Here's how to perform resistance band side leg raises:

1. Begin by placing a resistance band around your ankles. You can also place it just above your knees for a slightly different variation.

2. Stand with your feet together and your arms relaxed at your sides.

3. Engage your core for stability and balance.

4. With the resistance band in place, lift one leg out to the side as far as you comfortably can. Keep your leg straight and your toes pointing forward.

5. Hold your leg in the raised position for a moment, squeezing your outer thigh muscles.

6. Lower your leg back down to the starting position in a controlled manner. Don't let it touch the other leg or the ground between repetitions.

7. Perform the desired number of repetitions on one side, then switch to the other leg and repeat.

Here's a simple home workout routine using resistance band side leg raises:

Warm-up: Begin with a 5-10 minute warm-up that includes light cardio exercises and dynamic stretches to prepare your hip muscles.

Workout:

- Perform 3 sets of resistance band side leg raises for each leg.

- Aim for 12-15 repetitions per set.

- Rest for 30-60 seconds between each set.

Cool-down: After completing the side leg raise sets, cool down with 5-10 minutes of stretching exercises, focusing on your hip and thigh muscles.

Hydration and Recovery: Stay hydrated during your workout and after. Have a healthy post-workout snack or meal to support recovery.

Resistance band side leg raises are an effective exercise for strengthening the hip abductor muscles and improving hip stability. Proper form and control of the resistance band are essential to maximize the exercise's benefits and reduce the risk of injury. You can adjust the resistance level of the band to match your fitness level and gradually increase it as you get stronger.

Resistance Band Pallof Press:

The Pallof press with a resistance band is an effective exercise for strengthening the core and improving stability. It also engages the obliques and other muscles that help with anti-rotation. Here's how to perform the Pallof press with a resistance band as part of your home workout:

1. Begin by attaching your resistance band to a sturdy anchor point, such as a pole or a door frame. Make sure it's at chest height.

2. Stand sideways to the anchor point with your feet shoulder-width apart.

3. Grasp the resistance band with both hands and hold it at chest level. Your hands should be in the center of your chest, and there should be tension in the band.

4. Keep your core engaged and maintain good posture throughout the exercise.

5. Press the resistance band straight out in front of you, extending your arms fully. Keep the band centered on your chest.

6. Hold this position for a few seconds while resisting the band's pull to rotate you toward the anchor point.

7. Slowly return the resistance band to your chest, maintaining control throughout the movement.

8. Perform the desired number of repetitions on one side, then turn around and perform the same number of repetitions facing the other way.

Here's a simple home workout routine using the resistance band Pallof press:

Warm-up: Start with a 5-10 minute warm-up that includes light cardio exercises and dynamic stretches to prepare your core and stabilizing muscles.

Workout:

- Perform 3 sets of resistance band Pallof presses on each side (facing both ways).

- Aim for 8-10 repetitions per set.

- Rest for 30-60 seconds between each set.

Cool-down: After completing the Pallof press sets, cool down with 5-10 minutes of stretching exercises, focusing on your core and oblique muscles.

Hydration and Recovery: Stay hydrated during your workout and after. Have a healthy post-workout snack or meal to support recovery.

The resistance band Pallof press is an excellent exercise for core stability and anti-rotation. Proper form and control of the resistance band are essential to maximize the exercise's benefits and reduce the risk of injury. You can adjust the resistance level of the band to match your fitness level and gradually increase it as you get stronger.

Resistance Band Woodchoppers:

Resistance band woodchoppers are an effective exercise for strengthening the core, particularly the obliques, and improving rotational stability. Here's how to perform resistance band woodchoppers as part of your home workout:

1. Begin by anchoring your resistance band to a sturdy anchor point, such as a pole or a door frame. Make sure it's at shoulder height or slightly higher.

2. Stand sideways to the anchor point with your feet shoulder-width apart.

3. Grasp the resistance band with both hands, with one hand over the other and arms extended. Your hands should be at shoulder level.

4. Keep your core engaged and maintain good posture throughout the exercise.

5. Begin the movement by rotating your torso away from the anchor point while keeping your arms extended. Your hands should move diagonally across your body, simulating a woodchopping motion.

6. Pivot on your back foot as you rotate, and allow your hips to move naturally with your torso.

7. Continue the motion until your hands are at the opposite hip or slightly below it.

8. Reverse the movement and return to the starting position with control.

9. Perform the desired number of repetitions on one side, then switch to the other side by turning around and repeating the exercise in the opposite direction.

Here's a simple home workout routine using resistance band woodchoppers:

Warm-up: Start with a 5-10 minute warm-up that includes light cardio exercises and dynamic stretches to prepare your core and oblique muscles.

Workout:

- Perform 3 sets of resistance band woodchoppers on each side (facing both ways).

- Aim for 8-10 repetitions per set.

- Rest for 30-60 seconds between each set.

Cool-down: After completing the woodchopper sets, cool down with 5-10 minutes of stretching exercises, focusing on your core and oblique muscles.

Hydration and Recovery: Stay hydrated during your workout and after. Have a healthy post-workout snack or meal to support recovery.

Resistance band woodchoppers are an excellent exercise for core and oblique strength and rotational stability. Proper form and control of the resistance band are essential to maximize the exercise's benefits and reduce the risk of injury. You can adjust the resistance level of the band to match your fitness level and gradually increase it as you get stronger.

Resistance Band Shoulder Rotations:

Resistance band shoulder rotations are a useful exercise to improve shoulder mobility and strengthen the muscles that stabilize your shoulders. This exercise can help enhance flexibility and prevent shoulder injuries. Here's how to perform resistance band shoulder rotations as part of your home workout:

1. Start by anchoring your resistance band to a sturdy object at chest height, such as a pole or a door frame.

2. Stand facing away from the anchor point, grasping the band with one hand.

3. Step away from the anchor point to create tension in the band, and position your feet shoulder-width apart.

4. Keep your core engaged and maintain good posture with a slight bend in your knees.

5. Hold the band with your arm extended in front of you, palm facing down. This is your starting position.

6. Begin the rotation by moving your arm away from the anchor point and out to the side while keeping your elbow slightly bent.

7. Rotate your arm until it's parallel to the floor or until you feel a comfortable stretch in your shoulder.

8. Slowly reverse the movement and bring your arm back to the starting position in a controlled manner.

9. Perform the desired number of repetitions on one side, then switch to the other hand and repeat the exercise.

Here's a simple home workout routine using resistance band shoulder rotations:

Warm-up: Start with a 5-10 minute warm-up that includes light cardio exercises and dynamic stretches to prepare your shoulder and upper body muscles.

Workout:

- Perform 3 sets of resistance band shoulder rotations for each arm.

- Aim for 10-12 repetitions per set.

- Rest for 30-60 seconds between each set.

Cool-down: After completing the shoulder rotation sets, cool down with 5-10 minutes of stretching exercises, focusing on your shoulder and upper body.

Hydration and Recovery: Stay hydrated during your workout and after. Have a healthy post-workout snack or meal to support recovery.

Resistance band shoulder rotations are an effective exercise for improving shoulder mobility and strengthening the muscles that support your shoulder joint. Proper form and control of the resistance band are essential to maximize the exercise's benefits and reduce the risk of injury. You can adjust the resistance level of the band to match your fitness level and gradually increase it as you get stronger.

Cardio Workouts

Running in Place:

Running in place is a simple yet effective aerobic exercise that you can do as a part of your home workout routine. It's a great way to get your heart rate up, burn calories, and improve cardiovascular fitness. Here's how to do it:

1. Stand with your feet hip-width apart in a comfortable and stable position.

2. Begin by lifting your knees alternately, as if you are running, while staying in one spot. Start with a slow pace, and as you get more comfortable, you can gradually increase your speed.

3. Swing your arms in a natural running motion to increase the intensity and help maintain balance.

4. Engage your core muscles to maintain proper posture and provide stability.

5. Continue running in place for the desired duration of your workout.

You can modify your running in place routine to suit your fitness level and goals:

Workout Suggestions:

- Interval Training: Alternate between periods of running at a high-intensity pace and walking or jogging at a lower intensity for recovery.

- High Knees: Lift your knees as high as possible with each step for an added challenge.

- Butt Kicks: Kick your heels up towards your glutes with each step, engaging the hamstrings.

- Marching in Place: If running is too intense, you can march in place, lifting your knees with each step.

Here's a sample home workout routine using running in place:

Warm-up: Begin with a 5-10 minute warm-up that includes light cardio exercises to prepare your muscles and joints.

Workout:

- Run in place for 20-30 seconds at a moderate to high intensity.

- Perform 3-4 sets with 30-60 seconds of rest between each set.

- As you progress, increase the running duration or intensity.

Cool-down: After completing the running in place sets, cool down with 5-10 minutes of stretching exercises, focusing on your leg muscles and overall body.

Hydration and Recovery: Stay hydrated during your workout and after. Have a healthy post-workout snack or meal to support recovery.

Running in place is a versatile and effective cardiovascular exercise that can be a key component of your home workout routine, helping you improve endurance and burn calories. Adjust the intensity and duration based on your fitness level and goals.

Jump Rope:

Jumping rope is a classic and effective home workout exercise that provides a great cardiovascular workout, improves coordination, and can help with weight loss and overall fitness. Here's how to jump rope as part of your home workout routine:

1. Select the Right Rope: Choose a jump rope that's the right length for you. Stand on the center of the rope and pull the handles upward. The handles should reach your armpits. Adjust the length accordingly.

2. Proper Form: Stand with your feet close together and the rope behind you. Hold the handles in each hand, and make sure the rope is taut.

3. Swing and Jump: Swing the rope over your head and jump over it as it comes toward your feet. Keep your feet together and use your wrists to turn the rope. Land softly on the balls of your feet.

4. Practice Timing: The key to successful jumping is timing. Focus on finding a rhythm and start with a slow, controlled pace.

5. Keep Your Arms Close: Keep your arms close to your sides and your elbows bent at about 90 degrees.

6. Jump with a Straight Back: Maintain good posture with your back straight, shoulders relaxed, and core engaged.

7. Use Your Wrists: Most of the work should come from your wrists, not your arms. Avoid excessive arm movement.

8. Start Slow: If you're new to jumping rope, start with short sessions and gradually build up both duration and intensity.

9. Variations: As you progress, you can add variations, such as high knees, double-unders (jumping with the rope passing under your feet twice with each jump), or alternate foot jumps.

10. Safety: Make sure you have enough space to jump without hitting objects or people. Wear comfortable, supportive footwear to reduce the risk of injury.

Here's a sample home workout routine using jumping rope:

Warm-up: Start with a 5-10 minute warm-up that includes light cardio exercises to prepare your muscles and joints.

Workout:

- Jump rope for 30 seconds at a moderate pace.

- Rest for 30 seconds.

- Repeat for 3-5 sets.

Cool-down: After completing the jump rope sets, cool down with 5-10 minutes of stretching exercises, focusing on your leg muscles and overall body.

Hydration and Recovery: Stay hydrated during your workout and after. Have a healthy post-workout snack or meal to support recovery.

Jumping rope is a versatile and effective cardiovascular exercise that can be a fun and challenging addition to your home workout routine. Adjust the intensity and duration based on your fitness level and goals. It's a full-body workout that can help you improve your cardiovascular fitness and burn calories.

Basic Structure of a HIIT Workout:

High-Intensity Interval Training (HIIT) is a highly effective and efficient form of exercise that involves short bursts of intense activity followed by brief periods of rest or lower-intensity activity. HIIT workouts are known for their ability to burn calories, improve cardiovascular fitness, and enhance overall strength and endurance. Here's how to incorporate HIIT into your home workout routine:

1. Warm-up: Start with a 5-10 minute warm-up to prepare your muscles and joints. This can include light cardio exercises like jumping jacks, jogging in place, or dynamic stretches.

2. HIIT Work Period: Perform a high-intensity exercise at maximum effort for a short duration, typically 20-30 seconds. Choose exercises that elevate your heart rate and engage multiple muscle groups, such as burpees, high knees, squat jumps, or mountain climbers.

3. Recovery Period: Follow the high-intensity exercise with a brief recovery period, typically 10-20 seconds, during which you perform a low-intensity exercise or rest. This allows your heart rate to come down slightly.

4. Repeat: Repeat the high-intensity and recovery cycles for a set number of rounds, usually 3-5 rounds. Gradually increase the number of rounds as your fitness level improves.

5. Cool-down: After completing the HIIT intervals, cool down with 5-10 minutes of stretching exercises to promote flexibility and reduce the risk of injury. Focus on the muscles you worked during the HIIT session.

Workout Examples:

Here's a sample HIIT workout that you can do at home:
- Round 1:
- High knees (20 seconds)
- Rest or march in place (10 seconds)
- Round 2:
- Burpees (20 seconds)
- Rest or jog in place (10 seconds)
- Round 3:
- Jump squats (20 seconds)
- Rest or do a low-impact squat (10 seconds)
- Round 4:
- Mountain climbers (20 seconds)
- Rest or hold a plank (10 seconds)
- Round 5:
- Bicycle crunches (20 seconds)
- Rest or do slow, controlled bicycle crunches (10 seconds)
Hydration and Recovery:
- Stay hydrated during your workout and after.

- HIIT can be demanding, so listen to your body. If you're new to HIIT, start with shorter sessions and gradually increase the intensity and duration as your fitness level improves.

HIIT is an effective way to burn calories, boost cardiovascular fitness, and build strength, all within a relatively short workout time. It's a versatile form of exercise that you can customize to suit your fitness level and goals. Remember to focus on proper form and technique to reduce the risk of injury, and consider consulting with a fitness professional if you're new to HIIT or have any underlying health concerns.

Stair Climbing at Home:

Stair climbing is an excellent cardiovascular exercise that can be done at home if you have access to a staircase or a stair climber machine. It's an effective way to improve your cardiovascular fitness, strengthen your lower body, and burn calories. Here's how to incorporate stair climbing into your home workout routine:

1. Safety First:
   - Ensure that the stairs you'll be using are safe and well-maintained to prevent any accidents.
   - Wear appropriate workout attire and supportive footwear to reduce the risk of injury.
   2. Warm-up:
   - Start with a 5-10 minute warm-up that includes light cardio exercises like jogging in place or jumping jacks to prepare your muscles and joints.
   3. Stair Climbing:
   - If you have access to a staircase, you can climb up and down the stairs at a moderate pace for a set duration. As you become more advanced, you can increase the intensity by taking the stairs two at a time or increasing your speed.
   - If you have a stair climber machine, you can use it to simulate stair climbing. Adjust the resistance and speed to match your fitness level.
   4. Cool-down:
   - After completing your stair climbing session, cool down with 5-10 minutes of stretching exercises to promote flexibility and reduce the risk of injury. Focus on the muscles you worked during the stair climbing.

Workout Examples:

Option 1 - Time-Based Workout:

- Climb the stairs or use the stair climber for 20-30 minutes at a moderate pace.

- You can vary your speed or intensity during this time to challenge yourself.

Option 2 - Interval Workout:

- Climb the stairs or use the stair climber for 1-2 minutes at a high intensity (faster pace or higher resistance).

- Follow this with 1-2 minutes of lower-intensity recovery.

- Repeat this interval for a total of 20-30 minutes.

Option 3 - Stair Circuit:

- Create a circuit that includes stair climbing along with other exercises such as push-ups, squats, or lunges.

- Perform each exercise for a set duration (e.g., 1 minute) and then move to the next exercise without rest.

- Repeat the circuit 2-3 times.

Hydration and Recovery:

- Stay hydrated during your workout and after.

- Pay attention to your body's signals. If you're new to stair climbing, start at a moderate pace and gradually increase the intensity and duration as your fitness level improves.

Stair climbing is an effective and versatile form of exercise that can help you improve cardiovascular fitness, build lower body strength, and burn calories. It's a full-body workout that you can adapt to your fitness level and goals.

Bicycle Sprints:

Bicycle sprints are a challenging and effective home workout exercise that combines cycling with high-intensity interval training (HIIT). This exercise can help improve cardiovascular fitness, boost leg strength, and burn calories. Here's how to perform bicycle sprints at home:

1. Set Up Your Station:
- Use a stationary bike, a spin bike, or a regular bicycle on a stationary trainer if you have one. Make sure your bike is set up in a safe and stable manner.
- Ensure the bike is adjusted to your size and comfort.
2. Warm-up:
- Begin with a 5-10 minute warm-up to prepare your muscles and joints. Start with a moderate-paced cycling to get your heart rate up.
3. Sprint Interval:
- Pedal as fast as you can for a short duration, typically 20-30 seconds. This should be an all-out effort.
- If you're using a stationary bike, increase the resistance to make it more challenging.
- Focus on your leg speed and power during this interval.
4. Recovery Interval:
- Follow the sprint interval with a 30-60 second recovery period of slower-paced cycling. This allows your heart rate to come down slightly.
5. Repeat:
- Alternate between the sprint and recovery intervals for a set number of rounds, typically 6-10 rounds. Gradually increase the number of rounds as your fitness level improves.

6. Cool-down:

- After completing the bicycle sprints, cool down with 5-10 minutes of cycling at a moderate pace to gradually bring your heart rate back to normal.

Workout Suggestions:

- Start with a sprint duration of 20 seconds and a recovery duration of 40-60 seconds. As you get more experienced, you can increase the sprint duration or reduce the recovery duration.

- Focus on proper cycling form, keeping your back straight and your core engaged.

- If you're using a regular bicycle, make sure you're on a stationary trainer or in a safe and open space to perform these sprints.

Hydration and Recovery:

- Stay hydrated during your workout and after.

- Listen to your body, and if you're new to bicycle sprints, start with shorter sessions and gradually increase the intensity and duration as your fitness level improves.

Bicycle sprints are a powerful way to improve cardiovascular fitness, leg strength, and overall endurance. HIIT-style workouts, like bicycle sprints, can be efficient and effective for getting in a great workout at home. Adjust the intensity and duration based on your fitness level and goals.

Shadow Boxing:

Shadow boxing is a home workout exercise that involves throwing punches and moving around as if you were in a boxing match, but without a physical opponent. It's a great way to improve your cardiovascular fitness, build endurance, and enhance your boxing skills or general fitness. Here's how to incorporate shadow boxing into your home workout routine:

1. Warm-up:
   - Begin with a 5-10 minute warm-up to prepare your muscles and joints. Include light cardio exercises like jumping jacks, jogging in place, or dynamic stretches.
   2. Stance:
   - Stand with your feet shoulder-width apart.
   - If you're right-handed, your left foot should be forward (orthodox stance), and vice versa for left-handed individuals (southpaw stance).
   - Keep your knees slightly bent and your core engaged.
   3. Start Punching:
   - Begin with jabs (quick, straight punches with your lead hand) and crosses (straight punches with your rear hand).
   - Incorporate hooks (circular punches) and uppercuts (short, upward punches) into your routine.
   - Keep your punches controlled and focus on proper technique, extending your arms fully and pivoting on your feet for power.
   - Maintain a light bounce on the balls of your feet to simulate movement.
   4. Movement:

- Move around as if you're in a ring, circling your imaginary opponent and changing direction frequently.

- Use lateral and forward-backward movement.

- Combine punches with head movement, ducking, and bobbing and weaving to simulate real boxing tactics.

5. Combos and Defense:

- Develop punch combinations, mixing jabs, crosses, hooks, and uppercuts.

- Practice blocking and slipping punches as if you're defending against an opponent.

6. Intensity and Rounds:

- Shadow boxing can be done at different intensities. You can vary the pace, from a slow, controlled session to a high-intensity, fast-paced workout.

- Typically, shadow boxing is done in rounds, with each round lasting 2-3 minutes. You can start with 3-4 rounds and gradually increase the duration.

7. Cool-down:

- After completing your shadow boxing rounds, cool down with 5-10 minutes of stretching exercises, focusing on your upper body, legs, and overall flexibility.

Hydration and Recovery:

- Stay hydrated during your workout and after.

- Pay attention to your body's signals, and adjust the intensity and duration based on your fitness level and goals.

Shadow boxing is an engaging and effective home workout exercise that can help you improve cardiovascular fitness, build endurance, and enhance your boxing skills. You can tailor the intensity and duration to suit your fitness level and goals. It's also an excellent way to release stress and have fun while working out.

Dancing

Dancing is not only a fun and enjoyable activity, but it's also a fantastic way to get a great workout in the comfort of your own home. Dancing can help improve cardiovascular fitness, increase flexibility, and boost your mood. Here are some tips on how to incorporate dancing into your home workout routine:

1. Select Your Music:

- Choose music that you enjoy and that has a beat that motivates you to move. You can create playlists or use streaming services to find the perfect tunes for your dance workout.

2. Warm-up:

- Start with a 5-10 minute warm-up, which may include gentle stretches, light cardio moves, or simply dancing at a slow pace to gradually increase your heart rate.

3. Dance Styles:

- Experiment with different dance styles. You can try hip-hop, salsa, jazz, ballet, or any dance style that interests you.

- If you're new to dancing, you can start with basic movements and gradually incorporate more complex steps.

4. Dance Routine:

- Create a simple dance routine or follow along with online dance workout videos. Many fitness apps and platforms offer dance-based workouts with instructors to guide you through the steps.

5. Full-Body Engagement:

- Engage your entire body. Move your arms, legs, hips, and torso. Dancing is a full-body workout that can help improve coordination and balance.

6. Intensity and Duration:

- Adjust the intensity and duration of your dance workout to match your fitness level. You can start with a 15-30 minute session and gradually increase the time as you become more comfortable.

7. Cool-down:

- After your dance session, cool down with 5-10 minutes of stretching exercises to increase flexibility and prevent muscle soreness.

8. Variety:

- Keep things interesting by changing up your dance routine and music. You can explore different dance styles or try dancing to songs from various genres.

9. Dance Parties:

- Consider turning your home dance workouts into fun dance parties with friends or family members. Dancing together can be a great way to socialize and enjoy the workout.

10. Have Fun:

- The most important aspect of dancing is to have fun. Enjoy the music, move to the beat, and let yourself go.

Dancing is a versatile and enjoyable way to stay active at home. It's an effective cardiovascular workout that can help you improve fitness and boost your mood. Whether you're dancing to your favorite songs or following structured dance workouts, it's a great way to stay active and healthy.

Agility drills

Agility drills are a type of home workout that focuses on improving your speed, coordination, balance, and overall agility. These drills are especially useful for athletes who need to react quickly to changing conditions or for anyone looking to enhance their fitness level. Here are some agility drills you can incorporate into your home workout routine:

1. Ladder Drills:

- Lay an agility ladder (you can use chalk to draw lines if you don't have a physical ladder) on the floor.

- Perform a variety of footwork patterns, such as high knees, lateral shuffles, and two-foot hops, by moving through the ladder as quickly and accurately as possible.

2. Cone Drills:

- Set up cones or markers in various patterns and distances.

- Perform drills like cone weaves, T-drills, or 5-10-5 shuttle drills to improve your lateral speed, change of direction, and acceleration.

3. Dot Drills:

- Create a series of dots or markers on the floor in different patterns.

- Perform exercises like dot hops, dot drills, and dot agility circles to enhance your quickness, balance, and footwork.

4. T-Test:

- Draw a large "T" shape on the floor with tape or chalk.

- Start at the bottom of the "T" and sprint to the top, then shuffle left or right to the nearest leg of the "T," and finally backpedal to the starting point. This drill helps improve speed, lateral movement, and change of direction.

5. Box Drills:

- Use tape or markers to create a box on the floor.

- Perform box drills, such as the 4-corner drill, which involves hopping from one corner to another as quickly as possible.

6. Reaction Drills:

- Have a training partner call out directions, and react by moving quickly in the specified direction.

- This can include drills like the "mirror" drill, where you mimic your partner's movements, or the "chase" drill, where you react to your partner's movements by changing your direction.

7. Stair Drills:

- If you have access to stairs, use them for agility drills.

- You can do stair runs, lateral stair runs, or two-step stair runs to enhance lower body agility and cardiovascular fitness.

8. Hurdles and Obstacles:

- Use small hurdles, cones, or objects as obstacles to navigate around or over.

- Perform drills that involve jumping, stepping, and changing direction around these obstacles.

9. Mini Hurdle Drills:

- Place small, adjustable mini hurdles on the floor.

- Perform hurdle drills like lateral hops over hurdles or forward and backward hops.

10. Zigzag Runs:

- Set up a series of cones or markers in a zigzag pattern.

- Practice running through the pattern while changing direction quickly and maintaining balance.

11. Bear Crawls:

- Get into a bear crawl position (on hands and feet).

- Move forward and backward, crawl sideways, and change directions quickly to enhance agility and coordination.

12. Reaction Ball Drills:

- Use a reaction ball or a tennis ball.

- Bounce the ball and react quickly to catch it or hit it against a wall, improving your hand-eye coordination and reaction time.

When adding agility drills to your home workout routine, start slowly and gradually increase the intensity and complexity of the drills as you become more proficient. Agility training can be a valuable addition to your fitness routine, helping you improve your athletic performance and overall agility.

Creating a Workout Routine

Planning your home workout schedule is key to achieving your fitness goals, staying consistent, and making exercise a regular part of your life. Whether you're a beginner or a seasoned athlete, an organized and well-structured schedule can help you stay on track. Here are a few key principles to keep in mind when planning your home workout schedule:

- **Set realistic goals.** Don't try to do too much too soon, or you're likely to get discouraged and give up. Start with a few simple workouts and gradually increase the intensity and duration as you get stronger.

- **Find a workout routine that you enjoy.** If you hate what you're doing, you're less likely to stick with it. There are endless possibilities for home workouts, so find something that you find fun and challenging.

- **Make time for your workouts.** Schedule your workouts into your day just like you would any other important appointment. If you don't make time for them, they're likely to fall by the wayside.

- **Be flexible.** Life happens, and there will be days when you can't stick to your workout schedule. That's okay! Just do your best to get back on track as soon as possible.

- **Listen to your body.** If you're feeling pain, take a break. Pushing yourself too hard can lead to injuries.

● **Celebrate your successes.** As you reach your fitness goals, take some time to celebrate your accomplishments. This will help you stay motivated and on track.

Following these principles can help you create a home workout schedule that will help you reach your fitness goals.

Tracking your progress

Tracking your progress in home workouts is a vital aspect of achieving your fitness goals. Not only does it provide motivation, but it also helps you assess your performance and make necessary adjustments to your workout routine. One effective method to monitor progress is to keep a workout journal. Document the details of each session, including the exercises performed, the number of sets and repetitions, the amount of weight lifted, and the duration of cardio workouts. Over time, you'll see improvements in your strength, endurance, and overall fitness, which can be highly motivating.

Regularly taking measurements of your body, such as weight, body fat percentage, and circumference of various body parts, can also be helpful. While the scale is just one indicator, tracking changes in your body composition provides a more comprehensive view of your progress. Additionally, consider taking progress photos at regular intervals. These visual records can be remarkably motivating, as you can see the physical changes that might not be as evident day-to-day.

Another method to track your progress is to set specific, measurable, achievable, relevant, and time-bound (SMART) goals. These goals help you stay focused and committed, and they enable you to measure your success in a clear and objective manner. Regularly reassess your goals and adjust them as needed to keep your workouts challenging and rewarding. Remember that consistency is key to tracking and achieving your fitness progress.

Staying motivated

Staying motivated is key to sticking to a workout routine. To keep your motivation up, it's important to set clear and inspiring fitness goals. These goals should be specific, measurable, and achievable, so you have a clear direction and a sense of accomplishment when you reach them. Break down your larger goals into smaller milestones, and celebrate your successes regularly. Having a strong "why" behind your fitness journey, such as improved health, stress reduction, or weight loss, will give you a deeper source of motivation to keep you going.

Variety is another key to staying motivated. Trying different workouts, classes, or activities can prevent exercise from becoming monotonous. Explore new fitness challenges and keep your routine fresh and exciting. Additionally, it's important to have a consistent schedule for your workouts. Treat your exercise sessions as non-negotiable appointments, just like you would with any other commitment in your life. By scheduling your workouts and sticking to a routine, you create a sense of discipline and habit that will make it easier to stay motivated in the long run.contributes to your long-term motivation.

Positive self-talk and visualization techniques can also boost your motivation. Replace self-doubt and negative thoughts with positive affirmations that inspire confidence and determination. For example, instead of saying "I'm not good at this," you could say "I'm getting better every day." Visualization allows you to mentally rehearse your workouts and envision yourself successfully reaching your fitness goals. For example, you could picture yourself running a marathon or lifting weights. Remembering the numerous benefits of exercise, both physical and mental, can be a powerful motivator as well. Reflect on how good it feels after a workout, the increased energy, the reduced stress, and the overall sense of well-being that exercise brings. By embracing these strategies and staying committed to your goals, you can maintain the motivation needed to continue your fitness journey.

Here are some additional tips to stay motivated:

- Set realistic goals and track your progress.

- Find a workout buddy or join a fitness class.

- Reward yourself for your accomplishments.

- Make exercise a part of your daily routine.

- Don't give up if you have a setback. Just get back on track and keep going.

Nutrition and Recovery

Proper nutrition is the cornerstone of achieving and maintaining your fitness and health goals. Whether your objective is to build muscle, lose weight, improve endurance, or simply maintain overall well-being, the right nutrition plan is essential. To start, it's crucial to determine your specific goals and tailor your diet accordingly. For those looking to build muscle and strength, a diet rich in protein is key, while individuals aiming to shed excess weight may need to focus on calorie control and portion sizes. Your nutrition should be in alignment with your objectives to optimize your progress.

Incorporating a well-balanced mix of macronutrients is vital. Carbohydrates provide energy for workouts and should be adjusted to your activity level, while healthy fats support overall health. Protein, in the form of lean meats, dairy, or plant-based sources, helps repair and build muscle. Fiber-rich foods like fruits, vegetables, and whole grains are essential for digestive health and maintaining satiety. Hydration is also fundamental; staying properly hydrated ensures optimal bodily functions and can aid in managing your appetite and cravings.

Remember that portion control and meal timing are equally important. Consuming the right nutrients in the right quantities at the right times can make a significant difference. To truly customize your nutrition for your goals, consulting a registered dietitian or nutritionist can be beneficial. They can help design a meal plan that suits your specific needs and preferences, making it more likely that you'll successfully achieve and maintain your desired fitness and health outcomes.

Hydration is a fundamental aspect of maintaining overall health and well-being. Staying adequately hydrated is essential for your body to function optimally. Water is involved in various bodily processes, including digestion, circulation, temperature regulation, and waste removal. Without sufficient hydration, these functions can be compromised. Dehydration can lead to a range of health issues, from mild discomfort to severe complications.

Proper hydration is particularly crucial during physical activity and exercise. When you work out, your body loses fluids through sweat, which can lead to dehydration if not adequately replenished. Dehydration during exercise can result in reduced performance, muscle cramps, heat-related illnesses, and fatigue. To avoid these issues, it's important to drink water before, during, and after your workouts. The exact amount of water you need varies depending on factors like your activity level, climate, and individual body composition. A general guideline is to drink at least 8-10 cups (64-80 ounces) of water daily, but this can increase significantly during exercise.

A well-hydrated body also aids in weight management and appetite control. Sometimes, thirst can be confused with hunger, leading to unnecessary calorie consumption. By staying adequately hydrated, you can better distinguish between thirst and hunger, potentially reducing overeating and aiding in your weight management efforts. Proper hydration can also support healthier skin, improved digestion, and better cognitive function. To maintain optimal hydration, listen to your body's cues and consume water consistently throughout the day, not just when you feel thirsty.

Sleep and recovery are integral components of a healthy and effective fitness routine. Adequate sleep is vital for both physical and mental well-being, and it plays a crucial role in your body's ability to recover from exercise. During sleep, your body goes through a series of processes that help repair and rejuvenate muscles, consolidate memory, and regulate various physiological functions.

Physical recovery occurs during deep sleep stages, such as slow-wave and REM (rapid eye movement) sleep. During these stages, your body releases growth hormone, which is essential for repairing and building muscle tissue. Sleep also helps reduce inflammation and promotes the healing of minor injuries and muscle soreness that can occur during workouts. A consistent and quality sleep pattern is, therefore, a key factor in achieving optimal fitness results.

Sleep also plays a critical role in cognitive and emotional recovery. It enhances mood, concentration, and problem-solving abilities, which are important for maintaining motivation and mental resilience during your fitness journey. Inadequate sleep can lead to increased stress, irritability, and decreased tolerance for physical discomfort, potentially hindering your motivation to exercise. To support your fitness goals, prioritize sleep hygiene practices such as maintaining a regular sleep schedule, creating a comfortable sleep environment, and limiting caffeine and screen time before bedtime. By embracing good sleep practices, you can optimize your recovery, mental well-being, and overall fitness progress.

Workout logs

A workout log is a valuable tool for tracking your exercise routines, progress, and goals. It helps you stay organized and motivated in your fitness journey. Below is an example of what a workout log might look like. You can customize it to fit your specific needs and preferences.

—-

Workout Log for [Month/Year]
    Day 1: [Date] - [Workout Type]
    - Warm-up: [Warm-up exercises and duration]
    - Main Workout:
    - Exercise 1: [Exercise name] - Sets: [Number], Reps: [Number], Weight: [Amount]
    - Exercise 2: [Exercise name] - Sets: [Number], Reps: [Number], Weight: [Amount]
    - ...
    - Cool-down: [Cool-down exercises and duration]
    - Notes: [Any additional comments or observations]
    Day 2: [Date] - [Workout Type]
    - Warm-up: [Warm-up exercises and duration]
    - Main Workout:
    - Exercise 1: [Exercise name] - Sets: [Number], Reps: [Number], Weight: [Amount]
    - Exercise 2: [Exercise name] - Sets: [Number], Reps: [Number], Weight: [Amount]
    - ...
    - Cool-down: [Cool-down exercises and duration]
    - Notes: [Any additional comments or observations]
    Day 3: [Date] - [Workout Type]
    - Warm-up: [Warm-up exercises and duration]

- Main Workout:
    - Exercise 1: [Exercise name] - Sets: [Number], Reps: [Number], Weight: [Amount]
    - Exercise 2: [Exercise name] - Sets: [Number], Reps: [Number], Weight: [Amount]
    - ...
    - Cool-down: [Cool-down exercises and duration]
    - Notes: [Any additional comments or observations]
Day 4: Rest or Active Recovery
Day 5: [Date] - [Workout Type]
- Warm-up: [Warm-up exercises and duration]
- Main Workout:
    - Exercise 1: [Exercise name] - Sets: [Number], Reps: [Number], Weight: [Amount]
    - Exercise 2: [Exercise name] - Sets: [Number], Reps: [Number], Weight: [Amount]
    - ...
    - Cool-down: [Cool-down exercises and duration]
    - Notes: [Any additional comments or observations]
Day 6: [Date] - [Workout Type]
- Warm-up: [Warm-up exercises and duration]
- Main Workout:
    - Exercise 1: [Exercise name] - Sets: [Number], Reps: [Number], Weight: [Amount]
    - Exercise 2: [Exercise name] - Sets: [Number], Reps: [Number], Weight: [Amount]
    - ...
    - Cool-down: [Cool-down exercises and duration]
    - Notes: [Any additional comments or observations]
Day 7: Rest or Active Recovery
Summary for the Week:
- Total Workouts: [Number]

- Total Rest/Recovery Days: [Number]
- Achievements: [Highlight any accomplishments, improvements, or milestones]
- Goals for Next Week: [Set specific goals or targets for the upcoming week]

—-

This workout log allows you to document your daily exercise routines, including warm-ups and cool-downs, along with notes about your performance and how you felt during the workout. Reviewing your workout log regularly can help you assess your progress, identify areas for improvement, and adjust your fitness plan accordingly. It's a valuable tool for staying committed to your fitness goals and tracking your journey to better health and well-being.